BEI GRIN MACHT SICH IHR WISSEN BEZAHLT

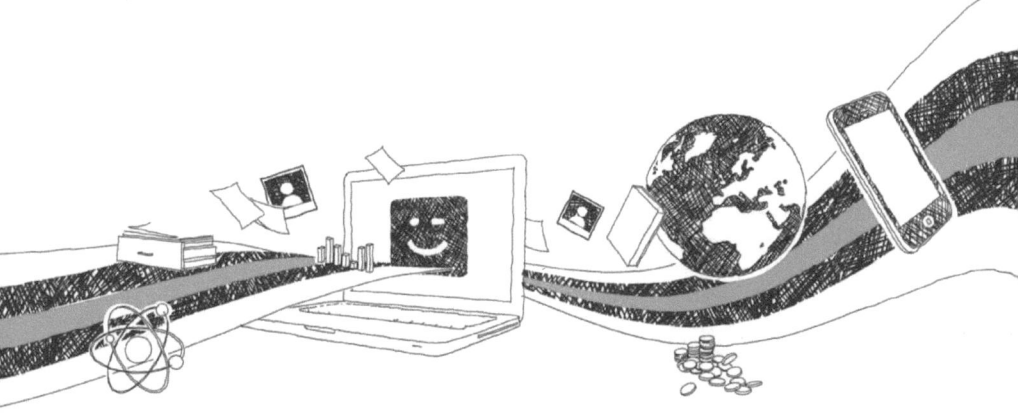

- Wir veröffentlichen Ihre Hausarbeit, Bachelor- und Masterarbeit

- Ihr eigenes eBook und Buch - weltweit in allen wichtigen Shops

- Verdienen Sie an jedem Verkauf

Jetzt bei www.GRIN.com hochladen und kostenlos publizieren

Dr. Peter Ubah Okeke

Seroepidemiology of Hepatitis B Surface Antigen in Pregnancy

Medical virology

GRIN Verlag

Bibliografische Information der Deutschen Nationalbibliothek:

Die Deutsche Bibliothek verzeichnet diese Publikation in der Deutschen Nationalbibliografie; detaillierte bibliografische Daten sind im Internet über http://dnb.d-nb.de/ abrufbar.

Dieses Werk sowie alle darin enthaltenen einzelnen Beiträge und Abbildungen sind urheberrechtlich geschützt. Jede Verwertung, die nicht ausdrücklich vom Urheberrechtsschutz zugelassen ist, bedarf der vorherigen Zustimmung des Verlages. Das gilt insbesondere für Vervielfältigungen, Bearbeitungen, Übersetzungen, Mikroverfilmungen, Auswertungen durch Datenbanken und für die Einspeicherung und Verarbeitung in elektronische Systeme. Alle Rechte, auch die des auszugsweisen Nachdrucks, der fotomechanischen Wiedergabe (einschließlich Mikrokopie) sowie der Auswertung durch Datenbanken oder ähnliche Einrichtungen, vorbehalten.

Impressum:

Copyright © 2012 GRIN Verlag, Open Publishing GmbH
Druck und Bindung: Books on Demand GmbH, Norderstedt Germany
ISBN: 978-3-656-28079-8

Dieses Buch bei GRIN:

http://www.grin.com/de/e-book/200500/seroepidemiology-of-hepatitis-b-surface-antigen-in-pregnancy

GRIN - Your knowledge has value

Der GRIN Verlag publiziert seit 1998 wissenschaftliche Arbeiten von Studenten, Hochschullehrern und anderen Akademikern als eBook und gedrucktes Buch. Die Verlagswebsite www.grin.com ist die ideale Plattform zur Veröffentlichung von Hausarbeiten, Abschlussarbeiten, wissenschaftlichen Aufsätzen, Dissertationen und Fachbüchern.

Besuchen Sie uns im Internet:

http://www.grin.com/

http://www.facebook.com/grincom

http://www.twitter.com/grin_com

SEROEPIDEMIOLOGY OF HEPATITIS B SURFACE ANTIGEN IN PREGNANCY

BY

PETER UBAH OKEKE

RESEARCH CONTENTS

Objectives..2

Abstract..3

Explanation of some abbreviations...4

Introduction...6

Literature review of HBsAg...14

Chemotherapeutic agents...18

Methodology...24

Results..27

Discussion...29

Conclusion..30

References..31

Appendix...36

Objectives

1. To study the occurrence of HbsAg among pregnant women in this locality.

2. To study the possibility of implementing routine HbsAg screening among pregnant women.

3. To study the classification of HbsAg of this locality into high, intermediate or low carrier status according to World Health Organization classification of HbsAg.

Limitations: α-fetoprotein assay, HBeAg and ultrasound scanning were not done.

Keywords: Epidemiology, Hepatitis B surface antigen, Pregnancy,

Abstract

A total of 83 pregnant women of Porto Novo were studied for HBsAg infectivity within the time period of 26th July to 30th August, 2012, during their first visit to the antenatal section- Hospital of Porto Novo. The age of the pregnant women studied range from 15 years to 46 years old.

The results of 1.2% were reported for HBsAg positivity among pregnant women of multigravid. They values of transaminase recorded at various stages were not statistically significant.

In conclusion, immunization of all infants, education of the general public and healthcare providers, and more research studies, among others, were advised for the elimination of hepatitis B virus infectivity in this region.

Keywords: Seroepidemiology, Hepatitis B surface antigen, Pregnancy,

Explanation of some of the Abbreviations used in this project

HBV: Hepatitis B virus, a double-shelled DNA virus of the Hepadnaviridae family.

HCC: Hepatocellular carcinoma or primary liver cancer- a major complication of chronic HBV infection; usually fatal.

Hep B_3: The third and final dose of Hepatitis B vaccine three doses are recommended for full protection.

Perinatal transmission: Transmission from mother to child at the time of birth.

Seroprevalence: Percentage of a population whose sera are positive for a specific marker such as an antibody, for example; anti-HBs or anti-HBc or an antigen, for example; HBsAg or HBeAg.

RNA: Ribonucleic Acid

DNA: Deoxyribonucleic Acid

AFP: α-fetoprotein

MHC: Major Histocompatibility complex

IFFCC: International federation of Clinical chemistry

Anti HBc: Antibodies against Hepatitis B core antigen

Anti HBs: Antibodies against Hepatitis B surface antigen, the presence of which indicates protection (either following infection or immunization)

Cirrhosis: Chronic infection and scarring of the liver as a result of chronic inflammation of the liver.

Chronic carrier: Person with long-term HBV infection defined as persistence of HBsAg in the blood for more than six months.

Hep B: A liver inflammation caused by the Hepatitis B virus.

HBcAg: Hepatitis B core antigen, a protein found in the core of HBV.

HBeAg: Hepatitis B e antigen, the presence of which implies active viral replication, thus making it a marker of greater infectivity in chronic infection.

HBsAg: Hepatitis B surface antigen; a protein from the virus coat. Its presence in the blood indicates current infection (acute or chronic).

BCG: Bacillus Calmette Guerin (Vaccine).

DTP: Diphtheria-Tetanus-Pertussis (Vaccine).

EPI: Expanded Program on Immunization.

FIC: Fully Immunized Child.

HBIG: Hepatitis B immune Globulin.

Hib: Haemophilus Influenzae type b (Vaccine).

OPV: Oral Polio vaccine

SIGN: Safe injections Global Network.

VVM: Vaccine vial monitor.

Introduction to Hepatitis B surface Antigen

Hepatitis is a general term which means inflammation of the liver and this inflammation could be caused by different types of hepatitis; A, B, C, D and E. Of the many viral causes of human hepatitis, hepatitis B and hepatitis C are of global medical importance, Hollinger, FB et al (2001). The development of jaundice is a significant feature of liver disease; a laboratory diagnosis could be made by testing the patients' sera for the presence of specific anti- viral antigens or antibodies. Hepatitis B is a serious and common infectious disease of the liver affecting millions of people worldwide, Chisari, FN et al (1997). The severe pathological consequences of persistent HBV infections include; the development of chronic hepatic insufficiency, cirrhosis, and hepatocellular carcinoma. Furthermore, HBV carriers can transmit the disease for many years, Robinson, WS (1994).

Every year, there are over 4 million acute clinical cases of HBV, and about 25% of carriers, a million people a year dies from chronic active hepatitis, cirrhosis or primary liver cancer, World Health Organization (2001). Hepatitis B has been correctly called type B hepatitis, Serum hepatitis, Homologous serum Jaundice, Mahoney FJ & Kane M (1999).

Causes of Hepatitis B

Hepatitis B is caused by hepatitis B virus (HBV), an enveloped virus containing a partially double stranded, circular DNA genome and fall into the family, Hepadnavirus. The virus interferes with the functions of the liver while replicating in hepatocytes. The immune system is then activated to produce a specific reaction to combat and possibly eradicate the infectious agent. As a consequence of pathological damage, the liver becomes inflamed. HBV may be responsible for about 80% of all cases of hepatocellular carcinoma worldwide, only second to tobacco among known human carcinogens, (Viral Hepatitis Prevention Board, 1996).

Spreading of Hepatitis B Virus

The majority of the people infected looks perfectly healthy and have no symptoms at all. HBV is transmitted through percutaneous or parenteral contact with infected blood, transmission associated with injection and blood transfusion, body fluids, child to child, and by sexual intercourse, Gitlin N (1997). HBV is able to remain on any surface it comes into contact with, for about a week, example, table tops, razorblades, blood stains, blades used in local circumcision, used needles, without losing its infectivity. HBV is a large virus and does not cross the placenta; hence it cannot infect the fetus, unless there is a breakage in the maternal- fetal barrier. Still, pregnant mothers who are infected with HBV can transmit their disease to their fetus at birth. If these fetuses were not vaccinated at birth, many of them will develop life-long HBV infections and yet many will develop liver failure or liver cancer later in life. Sexual intercourse with multiple partners makes the person prone to a danger of contamination and HBV is the only sexually transmitted infection for which there is a protective vaccine, Mahoney FJ & Kane M (1999). All persons who are HBV positive are potentially infectious. The many millions of people around the world who become HBV carriers are a constant source of new infections for those who have never contracted the virus.

Perinatal Transmission of HBV

Perinatal transmission from mothers infected with HBV to newborn infants is a major way of HBV infection in some countries, Okada K et al (1976). This happens at the time of birth; in-utero transmission is relatively rare, accounting for up to 2% of perinatal infections in most research studies, Wong VC et al (1984). The danger of perinatal transmission depends on the presence of hepatitis B e antigen (HBeAg) in the blood of mothers infected with HBV. The risk of chronic HBV infection is in the approximate range of 70% to 90% from such mothers, who are HBeAg positive and about 5% to 20% from those who are HBeAg negative, Margolis et al (1997).

Child to child transmission

The spread of HBV from child to child accounts for most HBV infections, Martinson FE et al (1998). Transmission usually happens in household settings but could also happen in child day care centers and in schools. The mechanisms of child to child spread include; contact of skin sores, small breaks in the skin, mucous membrane with blood or skin sore secretions. HBV may also spread due to contact with saliva by bites or other breaks in the skin, Beasley & Hwang (1983).Furthermore, the virus may spread from inanimate objects such as shared towels or toothbrushes.

Transmission associated with injection and blood transfusion

Unsafe injection practices are a major source of transmission of HBV and other blood borne pathogens in many countries, Simonsen L et al (1999). Blood transfusion is a major source of HBV transmission in countries where the blood supply is not screened for HBsAg due to financial restraints. However, in many developing countries, up to 50% of injections are administered with needles and syringes that are reused without adequate sterilization. A substantial proportion of therapeutic injections, accounting for approximately 90% of the estimated 12 billion injections administered each year throughout the world are really unnecessary. Injectable medications given in primary care settings can be administered via oral, stated by Drs. Hutin & Chen (1999). Unsatisfactory injection control practices including the reuse of contaminated medical or dental equipment, failure to use appropriate disinfection and sterilization practices for equipment and environmental surfaces, and improper use of multidose medication vials can result in the transmission of HBV and other blood borne pathogens. Finally, the injection of illicit drugs is a common mode of HBV transmission in some countries.

Sexual transmission

HBV is efficiently transmitted by sexual contact, which can account for a high proportion of new hepatitis B infections among adolescents and adults in countries with low and intermediate endemicity of chronic HBV infection reported by Drs. Alter MJ & Margolis HS (1990). In countries where HBV infection is highly endemic, sexual transmission does not account for a high percentage of cases because persons are already infected during childhood.

Persons at risk

The general public is at risk. Only persons who have been vaccinated successfully or those who have developed anti-HBs antibodies after HBV infection are immune to HBV infection. Persons with congenital or acquired immunodeficiency, including HIV infection, and those with immunosuppression, including those with lymphoproliferative disease, and patients treated with immunosuppressive drugs and patients on hemodialysis are more likely to develop persistent infection with HBV. Following acute HBV infection, the risk of developing chronic infection varies inversely with age. Chronic HBV infection occurs among about 90% of infants infected at birth, 25 to 50% of children infected at 1 to 5 years of age and about 1 to 5% of persons infected as older children and adults, Robinson WS (1995).

Epidemiology

Globally, the world can be divided into three areas where the prevalence of chronic HBV infection is high (≥8%), intermediate (2 to 8%), and low (≤2%), Mahoney FJ & Kane M (1999). High prevalence areas are South- East Asian and the pacific Basin (excluding Japan, Australia and New Zealand), Sub-Sahara Africa, the Amazon Basin, parts of the Middle East, the Central Asian Republics and some countries in Eastern Europe. In these areas, about 70 to 90% of the population becomes HBV infected before aged 40 and 8 to 20% of people are HBV carriers, Hollinger FB (2001).

China, Senegal, and Thailand, infection rates are very high in infants. In some countries such as Panama, Papua New Guinea, Solomon Islands and Greenland, infection rates in infants are relatively low, but increase rapidly during early childhood. Low endemicity areas include; North America, Western and Northern Europe, Australia and parts of South America. The carrier rate here is less than 2% and less than 20% of the population is infected with HBV, Hollinger FB (2001). The rest of the world falls into intermediate range of HBV prevalence, with 2 to 8% of a given population being HBV carriers.

Life Cycle of Hepatitis B Virus

The HBV binds to a receptor at the surface of the liver and other receptors include, transferring receptors, the asialoglycoprotein receptors and liver endonexin. Although, the mechanism is not known, viral nucleocapsids enter the cell and reach the nucleus where viral genome is attached. In the nucleus, second strand DNA synthesis is completed and the gaps in both strands are repaired to yield a covalently closed circular supercoiled DNA molecule that serves as a template for transcription of RNAs.

These transcripts are polyadenylated and transported to the cytoplasm, where they are translated into the viral nucleocapsid and precore antigen (C, Pre-C), Polymerase (P), envelope-L (Large), Medium (M), Small(S) and transcriptional transactivating proteins (X), Mahoney FJ & Kane M (1999).

The envelope proteins insert themselves as integral membrane proteins into the lipid membrane of the endoplasmic reticulum (ER). The process of conversion of RNA to DNA takes place inside the particles. The new, mature viral nucleocapsids can follow two different intracellular pathways; one of which leads to the formation and secretion of new virions, whereas the other leads to the amplification of the viral genome inside the cell nucleus.

In the virion, assembly pathway, the nucleocapsids reach the ER, where they associate with the envelope proteins and bud into the lumen of the ER, from which they are secreted via the Golgi apparatus out of the cell. In the genome amplification pathway, the nucleocapsids deliver their genome to amplify the intranuclear pool of covalently closed circular DNA. The precore polypeptide is transported into the ER lumen, where it's amino-and carboxyl-termini are trimmed and the resultant protein is secreted as precore antigen (e Ag). The X- protein contributes to the efficiency of HBV replication by interacting with different transcription factors, and is capable of stimulating both cell proliferation and apoptosis.

The HBV polymerase is a multifunctional enzyme. The products of the P gene are involved in multiple functions of the viral life cycle, including a priming activity to initiate minus- strand DNA synthesis, a polymerase activity, which synthesizes DNA by using either RNA or DNA templates, a nuclease activity which degrades the RNA strand of RNA-DNA hybrids, and the packaging of the RNA pregenome into nucleocapsids.

Hepatitis B Virus Infection- Disease state

HBV infection manifests in different ways depending on the patient's age at infection and immune status and the stage at which the disease is diagnosed. During the incubation phase of the disease, (mainly 6 to 24 weeks), patients may present vomiting, diarrhea, anorexia, and headache, Jaundice, low grade fever and loss of appetite. However, in most cases, HBV infection produces neither jaundice nor obvious symptoms.

The asymptomatic cases can be identified by detecting biochemical or virus specific serologic alterations in their blood. These patients could become silent carriers of the HBV virus and also a reservoir for further transmission to others. Most immunologically competent adult patients recover completely from their HBV infection, but about 5 to 10% will not clear the virus and will progress to constitute asymptomatic carriers or develop chronic hepatitis possibly resulting in cirrhosis or liver cancer. Rarely, others may progress to fulminant hepatitis and die. Furthermore, the frequency of clinical disease increases with age, whereas the percentage of carriers decreases with age. Globally, about a million deaths are recorded each year due to chronic forms of the disease, Viral Hepatitis prevention Board (1997). Persistent or chronic HBV infection is among the most common persistent viral diseases in humans. More than 350 million people in the world today are estimated to be persistently infected with HBV.

A large fraction of them are in Eastern Asia and Sub-Sahara Africa, where the associated complications of chronic liver disease and liver cancer are the most important health problems. A small number of long- established chronic carriers apparently terminate their active infection and become HBsAg-Negative, about 2% per year. Those who survive fulminant hepatitis rarely become infected persistently and HBsAg carriers frequently have no history of recognized acute hepatitis.

Acute hepatitis B infection- Clinical phases of infection

The acute form of the disease sometimes resolves simultaneously after few weeks of illness. Most patients recover completely without any consequences and without future recurrence of the disease. However, in geriatric population, a favorable prognosis is not feasible and can develop to fulminating and fatal acute hepatic necrosis. In pediatric population development to acute clinical disease is rare, but many of those infected before the age of seven will become chronic carriers, Robinson WS (1994). The incubation period varies usually between 45 and 120 days, with an average of 60 to 100 days. The variation is related to the infective dose of the virus, the mode of infectivity and host factors.

The hallmark of acute viral hepatitis is the striking elevation in serum transaminase activity. The increase in aminotransferases, especially Alanine aminotransferase (ALT), during the acute hepatitis B varies from a mild to moderate increase of 3 to 10 fold to a striking increase of more than 100 fold. The icteric phase of acute viral hepatitis usually begins within 10 days of the initial symptoms with the appearance of dark colour of urine followed by pale stools and of course yellowish discolouration of the mucous membrane, conjunctivae, sclera, and skin. Jaundice becomes apparent clinically, when the total bilirubin level exceeds 20mg/dl to 40mg/dl. It could be accompanied by hepatomegaly and splenomegaly. About 4 to 12 weeks thereafter, depending on immunogenicity, the jaundice disappears and the illness resolves, this can be seen in about 95% of cases in adults, Hollinger FB & Liang TJ (2001).

The larger the virus dose (infective dose), the shorter the incubation period becomes and the more likely it becomes for the patient to develop icteric hepatitis. The largest virus dose received by patients occurred in blood transfusion of infected blood, Robinson WS (1995). In most cases, no special therapy or diet is needed and the patients should not be isolated or confined to bed. Acute hepatitis B is characterized by the presence of anti- HBc Igm serum antibodies converting to IgG with convalescence and recovery, and the transient presence of HBsAg, HBeAg, and viral DNA, with clearance of these markers followed by seroconversion to anti- HBsAg and anti-HBeAg. Greater than 90% of adult onset infection cases fall into this category. The remaining 5 to 10% of adult onset infection and greater than 90% of cases of neonatal infection become chronic and might continue for the rest of the life of the patient. A small percentage of individuals die from acute HBV.

Chronic Hepatitis B infection

Although most adult patients recover completely from an acute episode of hepatitis B, but in a significant proportion, 5 to 10% of the virus persists in the body. In children, about 70 to 90% of infants infected in their first few years of life become chronic carriers of HBV. Chronic hepatitis can cause serious destructive disease of the liver and it contributes greatly to the burden of the disease globally and develops over many years during which patients will pass through a number of disease states. Surprisingly, some of these patients infected chronically may have no clinical or biochemical evidence of liver disease, while others may show signs of easy fatigability, anxiety, anorexia and malaise. Chronic hepatitis B is a prolonged infection with persistent serum levels of HBsAg and IgG anti-HBeAg and the absence of an anti-HBsAg antibody response. HBV DNA and HBeAg are often detectable at high concentrations, but may disappear if viral replication ceases or if mutations occur that prevents the synthesis of viral precore protein precursor of HBeAg. The associated inflammatory liver disease is variable in severity. It is always much milder than in acute Hepatitis B, but it can last for decades and proceed to cirrhosis and it is associated with a 100 fold increase in the risk of developing a hepatocellular carcinoma.

Three phases of viral replication occur during the period of HBV infection, especially in patients with chronic hepatitis B, Gitlin N (1997).

High replicative Phase: In this phase, HBsAg, HBeAg and HBV DNA are present and detectable in the sera or plasma. The risk of evolving to cirrhosis is very high.

Low replicative phase: This is when there is loss of HBeAg or a decrease or also loss of the HBV DNA concentrations. There is a decreased propensity for inflammatory activity in the liver and serologic changes like the loss of HBV DNA and HBeAg are referred to as seroconversion.

Non- replicative phase: In this marker, viral replications are either absent or below detection level and the inflammation are drastically reduced although, if cirrhosis has already developed, it persists indefinitely.

In cirrhosis, liver cells die and are progressively replaced with fibrotic tissue leading to nodule formation. The internal structure of the liver is damaged leading to the obstruction of blood flow and decrease in liver function. This damage is attributed to recurrent immune responses stimulated by the presence of the virus. Because there is totally no symptoms associated with liver inflammation, progression of inflammation to cirrhosis can occur without the patient knowing it. Therefore most carriers continue to be contagious while some are not, depending on the presence of HBV DNA concentration of each one. A number of HBV patients with chronic hepatitis will develop hepatocellular carcinoma (HCC). Only about 5% of patients with cirrhosis develop HCC, while about 60% and 90% of HCC patients have underlying cirrhosis.

Patients who develop HCC as a result of malignant transformation of hepatocytes have a mean 5 years survival rate of 25% to 60%. This depends on the tumour size, its resectability, and the presence or absence of α- fetoprotein (AFP). When serum AFP is increased in HBsAg carriers, HCC can often be diagnosed by liver scanning or ultrasound procedures at a stage when the tumour can be cured by surgical resection. This suggests that HBsAg carriers should have regular serial serum AFP assay and ultrasound examinations at 6 months intervals for patients above 40 years and also recommended to be repeated regularly for all HBsAg carriers with cirrhosis. Up to 80% of liver cancers are due to HBV, when HCC develops clinically, the disease is fatal and the median survival frequency of HCC patients is less than 3 months, but if diagnosed early, the cancer has an 85% chance of cure. Treatment includes surgery, hepatic irradiation and use of cytotoxic drugs.

Host immune response in HBV infection cases

There is little evidence that humoral immunity plays a major role in the clearance of established HBV infection. Cell mediated immune responses specifically those involving cytotoxic T- Lymphocytes (CTLs), seem to be very important in this clearance. CD8-Positive, class 1 Major Histocompatibility Complex (MHC) - restricted CTLs directed against HBV nucleocapsid proteins is present in the peripheral blood of patients with acute, resolving hepatitis B. These cells are hardly detected in the blood of patients with chronic HBV infection, suggesting that the inability to generate such cells may be due to their sequestration elsewhere. Also detected are CTLs against envelop glycoprotein determinants, that are CD4-Positive, class II MHC – restricted.

Primary infection leads to an IgM and IgG response to HBcAg shortly after the appearance of HBsAg in serum, at the onset of hepatitis. Anti-HBs and anti-HBe appear in serum only several weeks later, when HBsAg and HBeAg are no longer detected, although in many HBsAg- positive patients, HBsAg- anti-HBs complexes can be found in serum.

Hepatitis B surface Antigen in pregnancy – Literature review.

The work of Karim Rumi et al (1998) reported 85.7% among pregnant Bangladesh women were positive for HbsAg and infectivity rate was high with 30.2% positive also for HbeAg. Perinatal transmission of hepatitis B virus from infected mother to infant often leads to severe long-term sequel. According to Dr. Karim Rumi et al, infants born to mothers that show positive for both HbsAg and HbeAg have 70% to 90% chance of acquiring perinatal HBV infection, and 85% to 90% of infected infants become chronic carriers. Shiraki K et al (1977) stated that 25% of these carrier children will die of primary hepatocellular carcinoma or cirrhosis and the death usually occur during adulthood when familial and financial responsibilities are at utmost importance. Furthermore, most of neonatal infections are asymptomatic or clinically mild, they serve as a source of HBV infection to others in their families and communities, and many become carrier mothers themselves and perpetuate the cycle. The testing of HbsAg among pregnant women in 4 urban areas of the United States of America based on race and / or ethnicity by Dr. Gary Euler et al , demonstrated that white non-Hispanics were positive for HbsAg at 0.60%, blacks non-Hispanics at 0.97%, Hispanics 0.14% and Asians were positive at 5.79%. However, to ensure that all urban infants who are born to HbsAg – positive women receive appropriate preventive measures, health officials in urban areas of the United States were advised to use urban area epidemiology rates to ensure completeness in handling HbsAg cases in pregnancy.

8.0% of pregnant women tested based on variables of age, parity and HIV status were positive for HbsAg in Mali ,West Africa observed by the work of Brett Maclean et al (2012). However, due to high endemicity of HbsAg and lack of avenues for easy identification of risk factors, they advocated free maternal HbsAg screening and immunization of all infants born by HbsAg positive women within 12 hours of birth.

The experience of James A. Ndako et al (2012) reported 17.2% of positivity HbsAg in pregnant women of Bauchi state, Northern Nigeria. Pregnant women in their second trimester showed higher infectivity of 12.8% than those in the first trimester and third trimester respectively. Nigeria has been classified among the group of countries endemic for HBV infections. Currently about 18 million Nigerians are infected, many of these people may not be aware of the danger that they are carriers of this deadly virus and hence fail to seek appropriate and timely medical and / or diagnostic attention.

The Ethiopian research of Dr. Fisseha Walle et al (2008) identified 5.3% of Ethiopian pregnant women were positive for HbsAg. Their work history enlisted hypodermic needles, sharp materials and tattoo for cosmetics as major risk factors in the intermediate endemicity findings of HbsAg infection among pregnant Ethiopians. This called for educational awareness in traditional unsafe injections and harmful traditional practices in Ethiopian.

Another research findings of Ahizechukwu Eke et al (2011), expressed 8.3% of HBsAg positivity among pregnant Nnewi women of South east, Nigeria and in this research, multiple sexual partners, blood transfusion, dental manipulations, sharing of sharps/needles and local circumcision were not shown to be significant mode of infectivity or transmission, and maternal age, educational status and HBV infection do not co-relate.

Universal hepatitis B vaccination in infancy was implemented in Israel in 1992, but the recently arrived Jewish immigrants from Ethiopia are the group with the highest rate of HBsAg carriage in Israel (about 10%), Zamir C et al (1999).

They results of Dr. Luksamijarulkul et al (2002), revealed that the significant risk factors for HBsAg positivity in pregnancy were: A History of jaundice, tattooing and sharing articles with their husbands, such as toothbrush, a spoon or drinking glass. They emphasized that apart from giving HBV vaccination as preventive measures, health education for improving personal hygiene and sexual behavior must be intensified.

The Saudi Arabian government implemented a universal program on HBV vaccination to avoid early acquisition of infection in 1990. The work of Al-mazrou and co-workers (2004), conducted 12 years after the launching of the program to assess regional variation on HBsAg infection demonstrated 3% positivity of HBsAg in pregnancy. Although a drastic reduction of infectivity were noted, they implored that government should continue with the giving of the first dose of HBV vaccine at birth.

According to Onwuliri E et al (2008), on general seropositive screening in Aboh Mbaise District of Imo state, Nigeria, noted another alarming rate of 20.53% of the pregnant mothers screened were positive. The highest infectivity of positive samples, were observed among women that are multigravid (16.6%). Hence, Onwuliri et al advocated intensive and persistent HBV vaccination to be practiced by the health care providers in the area and all pregnant women will be strictly screened for HBsAg during early prenatal visit to the health centre and again when admitted for delivery. The work of Drs. Mbamara & Obiechina (2010) was in contrast to that of Onwuliri because their technical laboratory testing of pregnant women in Onitsha, Nigeria, presented 2.2% seropositivity for HBsAg in pregnancy. The Mbamara & Obichiena (2010) also observed that age, parity or sociodemographic or biological factors did not show a significant contribution to HBsAg infectivity and Onitsha, Nigeria, has an intermediate endemicity of HBsAg.

Dr. Biswas S C et al (1989) carried out a diligent research on pregnant women of Chandigarh, India and expressed 2.3% positivity for HBV, the presence of HBeAg in the mothers' blood system, enhances vertical transmission of hepatitis B virus infection to their babies, they implored.

Co- infection of Human immunodeficiency virus (HIV) with HBV affects change in number of infected people worldwide, Nelson M (2002). Among people infected with HIV, 70% to 90% have been observed to have HBV exposure, while 10% to 15% have recorded chronic HBV infection, Seattle Treatment Education Project (2002). However, very limited research information on co-infection status in Africa is available, and often conflictive and contradictory results were seen. Nevertheless, sub- Sahara Africa housed about 29.4 million HIV infected people, high HIV and HBV co-infection could be expected. In Kenya, Ogutu et al (1990), observed 78% of AIDS patients had an evidence of HBV exposure while Dao B et al (2001), registered 0.88% co-infection rate in Burkina Faso, pregnant women.

Professor Denis Edo Agbonlahor, a Medical Microbiologist and co-researchers (2004), worked extensively on HBsAg and HIV among pregnant women in Anambra, Nigeria and reported 0.7% co-infection rate. Hence, they concluded that the more educated a pregnant woman is, the less the infection of HBV becomes and age distribution was a significant factor in co- infectivity.

Dr. Bacq (2008) recommended that all infants born to pregnant women who are carriers of HBsAg must receive a serovaccination against this HBsAg by intramuscular injection and hepatitis B immune globulin (H-BIG, 100IU or 200IU) in two different sites in the first hours after birth. Vaccination then must continue according to the protocol in use. However, the combination of vaccination and H-BIG is very effective in preventing chronic carriage in children with efficacy more than 90%; some children may nonetheless become contaminated especially when the viral load is very high during pregnancy. A medical specialist must be consulted, when HBsAg is found in a woman during pregnancy and the family should undergo complete serologic testing.

The experience of Dr. Niesert et al (1996) in Germany, identified pregnant women with HBsAg at 1.4% positivity and some of these tested had not undergone antenatal screening Hence, supporting a need for routine screening of all pregnant women for HBsAg in Germany.

A comparative reading of ancient researchers and modern researchers on HBsAg infection among pregnant women displayed that, HBsAg infectivity has reduced significantly with intensive hepatitis B vaccination program. Various hepatitis B antigen educational projects, good sanitary measures, safe maternal delivery system, reliable laboratory diagnostic equipments, safe blood transfusion practices, safe disposable of sharps including needles used in hospitals and other safe medical manipulations, all have contributed immensely to the reduction of HBsAg infectivity. Worldwide, cases of HBV infection in pregnancy are reducing in most countries that adhere strictly to the measures of HBsAg vaccination among others.

The use of active and passive immunoprophylaxis to reduce the risks of perinatal transmission of HBV is well tolerated and accepted in clinical practice. Hepatitis B immunoglobulin (HBIg) given at the time of birth in combination with three doses of the recombinant hepatitis B vaccine given over the first 6 months of life has been up to 95% efficacy in preventing perinatal transmission, the risks of perinatal transmission of HBV increases as the mothers viremia load increases. In other words, if a mother's viremia load reduces at the time of delivery, the risk of perinatal transmission is also reduced.

Chemotherapeutic agents associated with Hepatitis B infection in pregnancy.

Seven therapies were approved by the United States of America Food and drug administration (FDA) for the treatment of hepatitis B. They includes; Interferon (both standard and pegylated), Lamivudine, Adefovir, Entecavir, Telbivudine and Tenofovir, Lok AS & Mcmahon (2009). These factors must be considered before therapy is given and they are; safety in pregnancy for mother and fetus, trimester of the pregnancy, safety in breast feeding, efficacy of the drug, its barrier to resistivity and duration of therapy. If pregnancy is contemplated in the near future, it may be prudent to delay therapy until after the birth of the child, Keeffe EB et al (2008). This technical approach requires a careful medical assessment of the degree of hepatic activity and fibrosis, using non invasive methodology. Interferon cannot be used in pregnancy but can be used in women of child bearing age for a determined period of 48 weeks and often results in clinical remission with HBeAg seroconversion, Lau GK et al (2005).

A planned pregnancy is preferable and may influence the choice and timing of therapy or potentially the timing of pregnancy. Marcellin P et al (2008) reported that treatment with tenofovir is preferable and safe because of its efficacy, high barrier to resistance and safe data available in pregnancy, while Lamivudine is the second agent that is also considered safe in pregnancy, has a high chance of emergence of resistant virus with prolonged therapy and now is no longer a first line agent in the non- pregnant category, (Antiretroviral pregnancy Registry, 2010).

However, a clinical case could be made for treatment of HBV infection during pregnancy, they associated risks, and benefits must be meticulously considered. They benefits of treatment appears to be most pronounced in most cases with high maternal viremia. In such occasion, treatment options should be considered, weighed carefully and must be discussed with the patient at the start of third trimester. Viable and efficacy treatment options are limited to lamivudine, tenofovir, and telbivudine, of these, lamivudine and tenofovir appears to be the therapeutic options with reasonable and considerable human exposure and safety data in pregnancy, Dr. Tran et al (2008).

However, no antiviral agent has been approved by the FDA for use in pregnancy, hence when a woman on HBV antiviral treatment becomes pregnant, a decision must be taken whether she could continue treatment or treatment be withdrawn immediately. Once again, the health of the pregnant mother and the fetus are brought into focus independently, from the fetus perspective, the major danger is the risk of exposure to medication during early embryogenesis and from the mother′s perspective, the major issue at stake is whether stopping or changing medication will adversely affect both short and long term liver disease outcomes. Furthermore, all HBV antivirals are inhibitors of either nucleoside or nucleotide polymerases, preferentially target the RNA- dependent DNA polymerase of HBV, they also interfere with replication of mitochondrial DNA and this could result in mitochondrial toxicity leading to the lactic acidosis syndrome, Fontana RJ (2009). Although, lactic acidosis syndrome is not common in adults, less is known about the potential propensity of mitochondrial toxicity in the developing embryo and toxicity may have adverse effects in organogenesis of the developing embryo.

The studies conducted by the antiretroviral pregnancy Registry and the Development of Antiretroviral therapy, reported that Lamivudine and tenofovir are still the two agents with the most invivo experience in the first trimester and appear to be safe and no significant difference was reported based on different trimesters. Laconically, these data are reassuring but it is important for health care providers to know that Antiretroviral Pregnancy Registry has its limitations. This is because the Antiretroviral Pregnancy Registry record defects identified at the time of birth and does not include long term follow up of fetus and other developmental anomalies that occur at the long term follow up, for example; cardiac, renal and neurologic defects were not included in their research procedure and were simply omitted.

Transmission of HBV infection and breastfeeding

Early research studies claimed that HBV transmission could occur through breast milk, and more recent studies have also confirmed similar rates of acquisition, regardless of whether infants were fed with breast milk or formula. Beasley RP et al (1975) before the availability of neonatal immunization, reported that the rate of acquisition of HBV were 53% in breast fed infants and 60% in formula fed infants born to HBsAg positive mothers. However, these data are limited because the high vertical transmission rates were confounded with the true rate of acquisition from breast feeding.

Hill et al (2002) a research procedure conducted after the introduction of immunoprophylaxis discovered the rate of infection in breast fed and formula fed infants at 0% and 3% respectively. Thus, current guidelines state that breastfeeding is not contraindicated in HBV infected mothers who are not on antiretroviral therapy whose infants receive immunoprophylaxis, Lok AS & Mcmahon BJ (2009). For mothers on antiretroviral therapy, breastfeeding is not recommended, according to pharmacological information, It has not been recommended that women breastfeed their infants while taking Lamivudine or tenofovir to avoid risking postnatal transmission of Human immunodeficiency Virus(HIV) type 1 infection, (Lamivudine, GlaxoSmithKline, 2009 & Tenofovir, Gilead Sciences,2010). However, from basic medical knowledge, it is known that Lamivudine and tenofovir are both excreted into the human breast milk, but little is known about the consequences of antiretroviral agent exposure in infants during breastfeeding.

Routine Infant Vaccination

The routine vaccination of all infants as an integral part of national immunization schedules should be given top priority as a management guideline. In countries that are of intermediate, high, and low endemicity of HBV infection, routine infant hepatitis B vaccination should be regarded as a top priority because the majority of chronic infections occur during early childhood. In a country of low endemicity, the majority of chronic infections are acquired among adolescents and adults but early childhood infections are still necessary in maintaining the burden of chronic infection. Most children who are infected have mothers who are not infected with HBV disease. Routine childhood immunization is also necessary in order to achieve optimal prevention of HBV infections acquired by adolescents and adults, because strategies targeting adolescents and adults risk groups have failed to control hepatitis B adequately. These immunization strategies for high risk groups have not been very successful because of the difficulty of immunizing persons in many risk groups before they initiate high risk behaviors and because of infections occurring among people with no identified risk factor.

Formulations

Hepatitis B vaccines are available in monovalent formulations that afford protection only against hepatitis B, and in combination formulation that protect against hepatitis B and other diseases(for example DTP – Hep B, DTP-Hep B+ Hib, Hib-Hep B).

Monovalent hepatitis B vaccine must be used for the birth dose, while combination vaccines that include hepatitis B vaccine must not be used to give the birth dose of hepatitis B vaccine because DTP and Hib vaccines should not be given at birth. Either monovalent hepatitis B vaccine or combination vaccines could be used for later doses in the hepatitis B vaccine schedule.

Immunogenicity and efficacy of immunization in children

Pre-exposure immunization: This is a course of three doses of hepatitis B vaccine and this induces protective levels of antibody to HBsAg (anti-HBs) in over 95% of healthy infants and children, when given in a variety of schedules; at 6 weeks, 10 weeks, and 14 weeks; at 2 months, 4 months, and 6 months; at birth, 1 month and 6 months, Apinall & Kocks (1998). Children who are responders to hepatitis B vaccine are protected against acute hepatitis B and chronic infection of HBV.

Post-exposure immunization: This begins at birth with either hepatitis B vaccine alone or with hepatitis B vaccine and hepatitis B immune globulin (HBIG). This has the power to prevent the spread of more than 90% of HBV infection from mother to fetus, Andre & Zuckerman (1994). They efficacy of giving recombinant hepatitis B vaccines alone is similar to that of giving hepatitis B vaccine with HBIG. The use of HBIG is not very important especially in countries where pregnant women are not screened for HBsAg. Optimum efficacy in preventing perinatal HBV infections is achieved when hepatitis B vaccine is given within 24 hours after birth. If the first dose is given in more than seven days after birth, protection against perinatal transmission is not practicable.

Presentation

Hepatitis B vaccines are available in liquid single-dose and multidose glass vials and in prefilled single-dose injection devices. The multidose vials generally contain two, six, or ten doses.

Dosage

The standard pediatric dose is 0.5ml. The quantity of HBsAg protein per dose that induces a protective immune response in infants and children varies with the manufacturer, but normally ranges from 1.5µg to 10µg, because of differences in hepatitis B vaccine production processes. For this purpose, there is no international standard of vaccine potency expressed in µg HBsAg protein and the relative efficacy of different vaccines cannot be assessed on the basis of differences in HBsAg content.

Administration

Hepatitis B vaccine is given by intramuscular injection in the anterolateral aspect of the thigh (infants) or deltoid muscle (older children). It can be given safely on the same day as other vaccines (for example; DTP, OPV, Hib, Measles, BCG, and yellow fever vaccine). It can also be given at any time before or after a different inactivated or live vaccine because inactivated vaccines such as hepatitis B vaccine generally do not interfere with the immune response to other inactivated or live vaccines, Centre for Disease Control and Prevention (1994). If hepatitis B vaccine is administered on the same day as another injectable vaccine, it is necessary to give the two vaccines in different limbs. The injection equipment used for hepatitis B vaccine is the same type as that used for all other Expanded Program on immunization (EPI) vaccines except BCG. Sterile injection equipment is a watch word for all injections and standard disposable syringes (1.0ml or 2.0ml) can be used but must be used once only and dispose safely after use.

Practices to avoid when giving hepatitis B vaccine

- Hepatitis B vaccine **should not be given in the buttock** as this route of administration has been linked with decreased protective antibody levels.
- Hepatitis B vaccine **should not be given intradermally** because it produces an inadequate antibody response in infants.
- Hepatitis B vaccine **should not be mixed in the same syringe with other vaccines** unless specifically recommended by the manufacturer.

Temperature of storage

The storage temperature for hepatitis B vaccine is 2 to 8°c. It is stable at least for four years from the date of manufacture if stored at this temperature range. Most hepatitis B vaccines are relatively heat stable and have only a small loss of potency when stored between 20°c to 26°c for up to a year and at 37°c for two to six months, Melnick JL (1995). However, in each case, the manufacturer's instruction must be strictly followed and hepatitis B vaccines must never be kept frozen.

Limitations

Hepatitis B vaccine protects only against hepatitis B, it does not protect against other types of hepatitis or other causes of jaundice. More than 95% of infants develop protective antibodies after three doses of hepatitis B vaccine. However, a small percentage of people are not protected after vaccination.

Long-term protection and booster doses

The studies of Harpaz R et al(2000) and that of Hadler & Margolis (1992) showed that infants, children, and adults who have responded to the three doses hepatitis B immunization series are protected from the disease for up to 15 years, even if they lose protective antibodies overtime. West & Calandra (1996) reported that long term protection depends on immunological memory which allows a protective anamnestic antibody response after exposure to HBV. Booster doses of vaccine are therefore not recommended, European Consensus Group on Hepatitis B Immunity (2000).

Hepatitis B vaccine is very safe, Mild transient side effects that may occur after immunization include; soreness at the injection site, fatigue, headache, and irritability and fever. These transient side effects start within a day after the vaccine has been given and lasts for up to three days. When hepatitis B vaccine is given at the same time as DTP vaccine, the rate of fever and /or irritability is not higher than when DTP is given alone, serious allergic reactions to the vaccine is rare.

Educational Training of Health care staff

Training for health care staff in both the public and private sectors is essential in connection with the introduction of hepatitis B vaccine into national immunization schedules. The health officers are responsible for handling and administering the vaccine and they are a major source of information for parents and other members of the public. The extra burden of new educational training can be minimized if the delivery of information on hepatitis B is integrated into existing training programs. Health care staffs that need training include EPI personnel, Medical Doctors, nurses, midwives, traditional birth attendants, Community health officers and administrators.

Training of health care staff should include:

- Hepatitis B and its consequences.
- Mode of HBV transmission.
- The risk group factor.
- They efficacy of hepatitis B immunization.
- Limitations of hepatitis B vaccine.
- The target group or groups for immunization and why they are chosen.
- Handling and administration of the vaccine.
- Safe injection practices
- How to logically respond to parents questions about the vaccine.
- The importance of administering the first dose as soon as possible after birth to prevent perinatal HBV transmission.
- Methods for monitoring and evaluating the impact of hepatitis B immunization.

Methodology

Eighty-three (83) blood samples from pregnant women attending antenatal clinic (ANC) for the first visit, at Hospital Porto Novo were bled, taking note of their age, parity, and trimester of each pregnant women. Their various cards for ANC were marked with a letter (T) to avoid testing the same person again. The period for blood collection started on 26th July, 2012 to 30th August, 2012, all blood samples obtained were analyzed at the Pathology laboratory section of the Hospital Porto Novo, all the samples were tested for HBsAG (using Bioline, one step assay), Biochemical tests of Alanine Aminotransferase (ALAT) and Aspartate Aminotransferase (ASAT) were done using system of enzyme kinetics of Human- Germany. Positive sample(s) were subjected to Enzyme linked immunosorbent assay (ELISA) at the Hospital Dr. Baptista Sousa, Saõ Vicente, Cape Verde.

Technique

One step Bioline SD HBsAg test produced by standard diagnostic, Inc, Korea.

Explanation of the technique

The SD Bioline HBsAg test is an in-vitro immunochromatographic, one step assay designed for qualitative determination of HBsAg in human serum or plasma. This test cassette contains a membrane strip, which is precoated with mouse monoclonal anti-HBs capture antibody on test band region. The mouse monoclonal anti-HBs colloid gold conjugate and serum sample moves along the membrane chromatographically to the test region (T) and forms a visible line as the antibody-antigen- antibody gold particles complex forms. The SD Bioline HBsAg test cassette has a letter of T and C as Test line and control line on the surface of the cassette. Both the test line and control line in result window are not visible before applying any sample. The control line is used for procedural control. Control line should always appear if the test procedure is performed properly and the reagents of control line are working. The SD Bioline HBsAg can identify HBsAg in plasma or serum specimens with a 100% degree of sensitivity and specificity, below is the systematic representation of test procedure using one step Bioline.

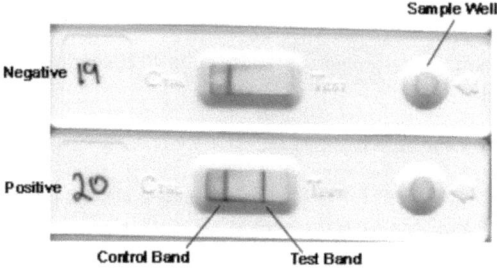

Alanine Aminotransferase -GPT (ALAT)

Alanine Aminotransferase (ALAT) kinetic method for the determination of ALAT activity produced by Human Diagnostics Worldwide, Germany, were performed according to the recommendations of the expert panel of the International Federation of clinical chemistry (IFCC). The reagents are ready for use and stable, even after opening, up to the stated expiry date, when protected from light at $2°c$ to $8°c$ and avoid contamination. The test can be performed at both room temperature $25°c$ to $30°c$, and at $37°c$.

Pipetting Procedure

Pipette into cuvettes	$25°c$ to $30°c$	$37°c$
Sample	200µl	100µl
Working reagent	1000µl	1000µl
Mix, read the absorbance after 1 minute and at the same time start the stop watch. Read the absorbance again exactly after 1, 2 and 3 minutes.		

Reading of results is automatic using our Humalyser 3000 system.

All Women blood samples performed at $37°c$ is up to **42 U/L** local reference range at laboratory Porto Novo.

Quality Control

All quality control Pathological and normal were done using Humatrol based animal serum provided with the reagent.

Aspartate Aminotransferase- GOT (ASAT)

This kinetic method for the determination of ASAT activity was according to the IFCC. The reagents were ready for use and stable after opening, once protected from light, stored at $2°c$ to $8°c$ and avoid contamination. The test can be performed at room temperature ($25°c$ to $30°c$), and also at $37°c$. The technical procedure is the same as that of the GPT (ALAT) above.

All Women blood samples performed at $37°c$ are up to **40 U/L** local reference range at laboratory Porto Novo.

Quality control is the same as that of GPT (ALAT).

Active hepatocellular damage is reflected by increased plasma levels of aspartate transaminase (AST) and alanine transaminase (ALT). In general, somewhat higher values of plasma alanine transaminase, which is solely cytoplasmic, than of aspartate transaminase (cytoplasm and mitochondrial) are found in acute viral hepatitis when cell membrane damage predominates. In viral hepatitis, the transaminase rises above normal during the prodromal period. Peak values of about 500 U/L to 2000 U/L are found at the time of maximum illness and the value returns to normal in about four weeks unless sub-acute liver disease develops, when levels become persistently elevated.

A similar but less marked increase with values rarely above 300 U/L usually occurs in non- icteric hepatitis and in glandular fever. Hepatocellular damage attributed to drug hypersensitivity may be shown by a continuing rise in plasma transaminase on repeated testing following administration of the drug. Alcohol raises the plasma transaminase levels in alcoholics but not in normal healthy subjects. Moderately raised plasma transaminase values usually between 50 to 300U/L are found in cirrhosis in proportion to the degree of active cell damage, but unrelated to coma or loss of liver cell mass. In malignant disease involving the liver, and in obstructive jaundice, the plasma transaminase values are usually moderately raised owing to Hepatocellular damage but rarely exceed 300 U/L. AST is also found in myocardium, being raised in myocardial infarction or following open cardiac surgery and in erythrocytes, being raised in autoimmune or invitro hemolysis. Destruction of large amounts of skeletal muscles as following road traffic accidents may also release the enzyme causing raised plasma levels. In these circumstances, it is unsuitable in the diagnosis or monitoring of liver disease.

Results

Age in years	Number, n (%)	HBsAg Positive (%)	HBsAg Negative (%)	Mean GOT U/L	Mean GPT U/L
15-25	50(60.24)	-	60.24	27.8	23.4
26-35	25(30.12)	4	28.92	28.4	21.6
36-46	8(9.64)	-	9.64	26.4	17.3

Table 1: Presented the overall distribution of HBsAg among all the pregnant women studied in relation to age (in years) and mean transaminase values (U/L) in September 2012, research work.

Gestational Trimester	HBsAg Positive n (%)	HBsAg Negative n (%)	Total (n)
First trimester	1(3.0)	32(38.6)	33
Second trimester	0(0)	19(23.0)	19
Third trimester	0(0)	31(37.3)	31

Table 2: Showed the distribution of HBsAg among pregnant women in relation to gestational trimester in September 2012, research project.

Parity status	Number n (%)	HBsAg Positive (%)	HBsAg Negative (%)
Primgravid	46	-	55.4
Multigravid	37	2.7	43.4
Total	83	1.2	98.8

Table 3: Presented the distribution of HBsAg of the pregnant women based on parity status in September 2012, research project.

Gestational trimester	Mean GOT U/L	Mean GPT U/L
First trimester	25.8	20.9
Second trimester	26.7	22.5
Third trimester	30.6	23.3

Table 4: Expressed the mean values of transaminase and its relationship to the gestational trimester of all the samples of the pregnant women in September 2012, research studies in Cape Verde.

Discussion

The HBsAg research studies conducted on 83 pregnant women of Porto Novo, Cape Verde, showed that 1.2% of those studied were positive for HBsAg among multigravid. The pregnant women that are primgravid among those studied were 55.4% while those who were multigravid were 44.6%. The pregnant women based on trimesters were thus; First trimesters were 39.8%, second trimesters were 22.9% and those who constituted third trimesters were 37.3% respectively. The age classification of pregnant women also showed that age 15 years to 25 years old were 60.24%, those that are up to 35 years were 30.12% and pregnant women more than 36 years old but not exceed 46 years old were 9.64%. The transaminase values recorded at various stages were not statistically significant, but transaminase values seem to increase with the increasing trimester as was observed in table 4 of the result presentation.

The infection of HBsAg in this locality is of low endemicity in line with the World Health Organization classification of HBsAg infection. The immunization of all infants born in Cape Verde with HBIG and /or HBV vaccine started in 2002, and this may have contributed to the control of HBV infection in this region and thus, could also contribute to the result recorded in this work. All infants born in this country were vaccinated at birth and subsequently follow the national protocol of vaccination in use here till the age of 18 months; most of these protocols contain HBV vaccine re-enforcement.

This research finding agreed with that obtained in most developed and developing countries, the work of Dr. Niesert et al (1996) reported 1.4% positivity for HBsAg among pregnant German women and that of Dr. Biswas et al (1989) recorded 2.2% of HBsAg positive among Indian pregnant women, also Mbamara & Obichiena (2010) observed 2.2% HBsAg positive among pregnant women in Onitsha, South-east Nigeria, Of all these, the studies conducted in Porto Novo is totally in agreement.

However, the work of Karim Rumi et al (1998) of 85.7% positivity for HBsAg among Bangladesh pregnant women, that of Dr. Brett Maclean et al (2012) of 8.0% positive for HBsAg among pregnant women of Mali- West Africa were totally in contrast compared to the studies of 1.2% positive for HBsAg obtained in Porto Novo.

The intensive educative program of the ministry of health, Cape Verde on HBV vaccination protocol, and the efforts of the health officers in charge of vaccination to ensure that every Capeverdian child is vaccinated is obvious as noted in this work. The studies conducted here will serve as a base for other workers, who could work on Praia city or Mindelo city, to do more by covering more pregnant population.

Conclusion

- ❖ Immunization, the most effective and cost saving means of prevention must continue.
- ❖ More research is needed to cover more pregnant women.
- ❖ Education of high risk groups and health care workers is necessary to reduce the risk of contracting the virus, thereby reducing the chances for transmission and to promote acceptance of vaccination protocol in use in Cape Verde.
- ❖ Any unscreened blood and /or its products must never be transfused.
- ❖ Monitoring of HBV infection incidence in Cape Verde must be effected and serological quality of tests used in Laboratories is crucial for firm diagnosis.
- ❖ Ministry of health must ensure adequate provision of laboratory reagents for HBsAg screening in the country.
- ❖ Efforts should be made for doctors to report all cases of jaundice and request laboratory tests as appropriate, surveillance reports should be submitted on regular basis.

References

Ahizechukwu Eke et al (2011): Prevalence, correlates and pattern of hepatitis B surface antigen in a low resource setting. Virology Journal 8 (12) Doi: 10 1186/1743-422X-8-12.

Al-Mazrou Y T et al (2004): Screening of pregnant Saudi women for hepatitis B surface antigen. Ann Scandi Med 24 (4): 265-269.

Alter MJ & Margolis HS (1990): The emergency of hepatitis B as a sexually transmitted disease. Med Clin North America 74:1529-1541.

Andre FE & Zuckerman AJ (1994): Review: Protective efficacy of hepatitis B vaccine in neonates. Journal of medical Vieology 44:144-151.

Antiretroviral Pregnancy Registry, http//www.apregistry.com

Apinall S & Kocks DJ (1998): Immunogenicity of a low- cost hepatitis B vaccine in the South African expanded Program on immunization. South African medical Journal 88:36.

Bacq Y (2008): Hepatitis B and Pregnancy. Gastroenterol Clin Biol 32 (1pt2):S12-9

Beasley RP & Hwang LT (1983): Postnatal infectivity of hepatitis B surface antigen carrier mothers. Journal of infectious Diseases 147:185.

Beasley RP et al (1975): Evidence against breast feeding as a mechanism for vertical transmission of Hepatitis B. Lancet 2: 740-741.

Biswas S C et al (1989): Prevalence of hepatitis B surface antigen in pregnant mothers and its perinatal transmission. Transac R Soc Trop. Med & Hyg 83 (5):698-700.

Brett Maclean et al (2012): Seroprevalence of Hepatitis B surface antigen among pregnant women attending the Hospital for women & children in Koutiala, Mali. South Afr Med J 102(1):47-49.

Centers for Disease Control and Prevention (1994): General recommendation on immunization: recommendation of the Advisory committee on immunization practices (ACIP). Morbidity and Mortality weekly report 43 (No. RR1):14-15.

Chisari F V & Ferrari C (1997): Viral Hepatitis. In: Nathanson N e tal eds. Viral pathogenesis. Philadelphia, Lippincott- Raven: 745-778.

Collenberg E et al (2006): Seroprevalence of six different viruses among pregnant women and bllod donors in rural and urban Burkina Faso: A comparative analysis. Journal of Medical Virology 78:683-692.

Dao B et al (2001): HIV infection and HBV co-infection: Survey of prevalence in pregnant women in Burkina Faso. Rev. Med. Brux, 2: 83-86.

Denis Agbonlahor, E et al (2004): The seroprevalence of Hepatitis B surface antigen and Human immunodeficiency virus among pregnant women in Anambra state, Nigeria. Department of internal medicine, Shiraz E- medical Journal Vol 5 (2):4

Erdem M M et al (1994): Prevalence of hepatitis B surface antigen among pregnant women in a low risk population. Int J Gynaecol Obstet 44(2): 125-128.

Eurler G L et al (2003): Hepatitis B surface antigen prevalence among pregnant in urban areas:Implications for testing, reporting and preventing perinatal transmission. Pediatrics 111 (5 part2):1192.

European Consensus Group on Hepatitis B immunity (2000): Are booster immunizations needed for lifelong hepatitis B immunity? Lancet 355:561.

Fisseha Walle et al (2008): Prevalence of Hepatitis B surface antigen among pregnant women attending antenatal care service at Debre- Tabor Hospital, Northwest Ethiopia. Ethiopia J Health Sc Vol 17(1):13.

Fontana RJ (2009): Side effects of long term oral antiviral therapy for hepatitis B. Hepatol 49: S185-S189.

Gitlin N (1997): Hepatitis B: Diagnosis, prevention and treatment. Clinical Chemistry, 43:1500-1506

Hadler SC & Margolis HS (1992): Hepatitis B immunization vaccine types, efficacy, and indications for immunization. In: Remington JS, Swartz MN eds. Current Topics in infectious Diseases vol12. Boston, Blackwell Scientific Publications: 282-308.

Harpaz R et al (2000): Elimination of chronic hepatitis B virus infections: results of the Alaska immunization program. Journal of infectious diseases 181:413.

Hill J B et al (2002): Risk of hepatitis B transmission in breast fed infants of chronic hepatitis B carriers. Obstet Gynecol 99:1049-1052.

Hollinger F B & Liang T J (2001): Hepatitis B Virus. In: Knipe D M et al, Eds. Fields Virology, 4th ed. Philadelphia, Lippincott Williams & Wilkins:2971-3036

Hutin YJF & Chen RT (1999): Injections safety: a global challenge. Bull. World Health Organization, 77:787-788.

James A Ndako et al (2012): Sero- survey of Hepatitis B surface antigen among pregnant women attending infectious Disease Hospital, Bayara, Bauchi state, Nigeria. Microbiology Research 3(1): 43.

Karim Rumi M A et al (1998): Detection of Hepatitis B surface antigen in pregnant women attending public Hospital for delivery: Implications for vaccination strategy in Bangladesh. Am J Trop. Med & Hyg 59 (2): 318-322.

Keeffe EB et al (2008): A treatment algorithm for the management of chronic hepatitis B in the United States. Clin Gastroenterol Hepatol 6:1315-1341.

Lamivudine: Research triangle park, NC: Glaxo SmithKline, 2009 at http://www.us.gsk.com/products/assets/usepivir.pdfl.

Lau GK et al (2005): Peg interferon Alfa-2a Lamivudine and the combination for HBeAg positive chronic hepatitis B. New England J Med (352): 2682-2695.

Lok AS & Mcmahon BJ (2009): Chronic hepatitis B. Hepatology 50: 1-36.

Luksamijarulkul P et al (2002): Risk factors for Hepatitis B surface antigen positivity among pregnant women. J Med Assoc Thailand 85(3): 283-288.

Magolis HS et al (1997): Viral hepatitis. In Evans AS, Kaslow RA (eds): Viral infection of humans. Epidemiology and control (4th ed), NewYork, Plenum Publishing: 363-418.

Mahoney F J & Kane M (1999): Hepatitis B Vaccine. In:Plotkin S A, Orenstein W A, Eds. Vaccines 3rd ed. Philadelphia, WB Saunders Company :158-182.

Marcellin P et al (2008): Tenofovir disoproxil fumarate versus Adefovir dipivoxil for chronic hepatitis B. Hepatol (359): 2442-2455.

Martinson FE et al (1998): Risk factors for horizontal transmission of hepatitis B virus in a rural district of Ghana. American Journal of Epidemiology 147:478.

Mbaawuaga E M et al (2008): Hepatitis B virus (HBV) infection among pregnant women of Makurdi, Nigeria. Afr J Biomed Res. 11:155-159.

Mbamara S U & Obiechina N J A (2010): Seroprevalence of hepatitis B surface antigen among antenatal clinic attendees in a private specialist hospital in Onitsha, South east, Nigeria. Nigeria Medical Journal vol 51 (4):152-154.

Melnick JL (1995): Thermostability of Poliovirus, measles, and hepatitis B vaccines. Vaccine Research 4:1-11.

Munderi P et al (2009): Pregnancy and outcomes among women on triple drug antiretroviral therapy (ART) in the DART trail. Fifth IAS conference on HIV pathogenesis, treatment and prevention Cape Town, South Africa, July 19-22.

Nelson M (2002): Updates on research studies on HIV co-infection with hepatitis B and C. XIV International AIDS conference, Barcelona, Spain July 7- 12.

Niesert S et al (1996): Prevalence of Hepatitis B in Pregnancy and selective screening. Geburtshilfe Frauenheilkd 56 (6): 283-286.

Ogutu E O et al (1990): The prevalence of HbsAg, antiHBs and antiHBc in patients with AIDS. East Afr Med J 65 (5): 355-358.

Okada K et al (1976): e antigen and anti-e in the serum of asymptomatic carrier mothers as indicators of positive and negative transmission of hepatitis B virus to their infants. New England Journal of medicine 294:746.

Onwuliri E et al (2008): Seroprevalence of hepatitis B surface antigen (HbsAg) among pregnant women in Aboh Mbaise Local district, Imo state, Nigeria. International Journal of Natural & Applied Sciences Vol. 4 Number 4

Robinson W S (1994): Hepatitis B Virus. General features Human. In: Webster R G, Granoft A eds. Encyclopedia of Virology. London, Academic press Ltd: 554-569

Robinson W S (1995): Hepatitis B and D Virus. In: Mandell G L, Bennett J E, Dolin R, eds Principles and practice of infectious diseases, 4th ed. New York Churchill Livingstone: 1406.

Seattle Treatment Education project (2002): Hepatitis co- infection: HIV/HBV co-infection. Issue, 3 (28), 1:36

Shirak K et al (1977): Hepatitis B surface antigen and chronic hepatitis in infants born to asymptomatic carrier mothers. Am J Dis Child 131:644-647

Sidibe S, et al (2001): Prevalence of serologic markers of the hepatitis B Virus in pregnant women of Bamako, Mali. Bull Soc Pathol Exot 94:339

Simonsen L et al (1999): Unsafe injections in the developing world and transmission of bloodborne pathogens: a review. Bull of the world Health organization 77:789-800.

Tenofovir DF: Foster City, CA: Gilead Sciences; 2010 at http://www.gilead.com/pdf/vireadpi.pdfl.

Tran T T et al (2008): Management of the pregnant hepatitis B patient. Current Hepatiti reports, 7:12-17.

Viral Hepatitis Prevention Board (1996): Prevention and control of hepatitis B in the community, Communicable Disease series 1.

Viral Hepatitis Prevention Board (1997): The clock is running, deadline for integrating hepatitis B vaccination into all national immunization programs.

West DJ & Calandra GB (1996): Vaccine induced immunologic memory for hepatitis B surface antigen: implications for policy on booster vaccination. Vaccine 14:1019.

Wong VC et al (1984): Prevention of the HBsAg carrier state in newborn infants of mothers who are chronic carriers of HBsAg and HBeAg by administration of hepatitis B vaccine and hepatitis B immunoglobulin. Double blind randomized placebo controlled study. Lancet 1:921.

World Health Organization (2001): Introduction of hepatitis B vaccination into childhood immunization services (unpublished report). Geneva, Switzerland.

World Health Organization (2002): Hepatitis B Virus, WHO, Geneva, Switzerland.

Wurrie I M et al (2005): Sero-prevalence of hepatitis B virus among middle to high socio-economic antenatal population in Sierra Leone. West Afr J Med 24:18-20.

Zamir C et al (1999): Evaluation of screening for hepatitis b surface antigen during pregnancy in a population with a high prevalence of hepatitis B surface antigen positive/ hepatitis B e antigen negative carriers. Pediatr Infect Dis J 18(3): 262-266.

APPENDIX

Routine vaccination in use in Cape Verde since 2010 is as follows:

- At birth or few hours after birth: BCG vaccine, Hepatitis B and OPV
- At 2 months : DTP, Hep B, Hib, (Vaccine Pentavalent) and OPV
- At 4 months: Vaccine Pentavalent and OPV
- At 6 months: Vaccine Pentavalent, and OPV
- At 9 months: Measles vaccine
- At 15 months: Parotidite, Rubella and measles (vaccine viral triplice)
- At 18 months: Vaccine Pentavalent, and OPV